Merriam Webster defines System as follows:
An organized or established procedure.

Now let's use it in a sentence.
The players loved the coaches' new system.

The system is written to serve as a foundational tool for living, to strengthen your commitment to self, to hold you accountable, and to assist you in living a healthy and active lifestyle.

Are you ready for the System?
Let's Go...

The Blueprint

The Challenge……………………………..Page 3

Phase I
Common Sense - The Process…………Page 5

Phase II
Project Management - The Model…Page 22

Phase III
Accountability – Ownership…………..Page 27

Phase IV
Health & Recreation - Keeping Active
………………………………………………………Page 33

Phase V
The Main Ingredient……………….…….Page 37

The Decision……………………….…..…..Page 38

The Challenge

Prior to reading this blueprint to a better life, one needs to ask themselves am I ready for this, am I truly ready to take on this magnificent transformation that is going to challenge me, hold me accountable, and test me each and every day of my life.

Again ask yourself am I up to the challenge, do I hold the intestinal fortitude to see this thing through from its inception to its fruition. Because if you don't I caution you, as this is going to be one of the biggest decisions you might ever make. So please take your time and maybe skim through the pages and feel the weight of the task.

After doing so, remember one thing it won't be easy, however it will be worth it, and it will mold you and take you to heights that you never could fathom. That is only if you take this as one of the most serious things that you have ever embarked upon. Really, are you ready? Then let's start

The System

Reading Objectives

1. Learn to ask Yourself, What's the Right thing to do? Then Choose Wisely. Learn to Embrace the Process.

2. Understand Why You Should Become Your First Project.

3. Understand the Importance of holding Yourself Accountable.

4. Understand the Importance of a Healthy Lifestyle

5. Find Your Main Ingredient

Phase I: Common Sense - The Process

Webster defines Common Sense as follows:
Common Sense - The unreflective opinions of ordinary people; sound and prudent but often unsophisticated judgment.

It defines Process as follows:
Process - The entire course of proceedings in a type of action (Life or Legal).

Folks have a tendency to shy away from common sense, as it usually suggest that you do the right thing. I say the sooner you adopt the common sense way of life, the sooner you will stop needing excuses for all of your failures. Through using common sense they will more than likely slow down, or possibly even come to a screeching halt. I know, it's tough because it keeps you honest, and in life you will be faced with plenty of opportunities to lie. Live by common sense and you won't need to lie, however you might find that your outcomes are far better than before. Try it.

Now with that said, we also need to know that in life there will come a process, and what we must learn to do, is trust it. Joel Embid of the Philadelphia 76ers said it best when his team was going through its rebuilding process. He said, and I quote him here "We as a team must learn to trust the process." You should know one thing about life, school, sports, the music industry, and to get 100% real world with you, even in the hustle game there will be a process. And one thing that remains true of all processes is that we must choose to either trust them, embrace them, or add to them. Basically, if we can't do either of these things then simply leave the process alone, as all we will end up doing is more than likely hurting or destroying it, and when this happens it will usually breed failure. On the other hand when the process is positive, and we learn to embrace it, that is when we become victorious. Victorious in life, school, sports, and most other areas where we decide to embrace the positive process.

Let's see what the folks at Wiki Now have to say about developing common sense:

How to Develop Common Sense

Common sense is the practice of acting intelligently in everyday situations. Even very smart people sometimes lack common sense, but luckily, it's an attribute that gets better with practice! By learning to reflect on a situation before you act, you can train yourself to use common sense before you make any decisions!

Quick Summary

If you want to develop common sense, start by mastering practical skills like learning to cook, budgeting your money, and repairing common household items. This will help you feel more connected to your environment, which can help encourage you to think practically about new situations which may arise. When you're presented with new information, try to analyze it with an open mind and ask questions rather than just accepting things. For more tips on developing common sense, like practicing rapid cognition, check out these steps.

1. Familiarize yourself with the purpose and meaning of common sense.

According to Merriam Webster, common sense is about exercising "sound and prudent judgment based on a simple perception of the situation or facts".[1] This definition suggests that common sense depends on not over-complicating the situation (simple), applying experience and general knowledge to the situation (sound and prudent judgment), and implicit in this is self-trust that your considered experience is valid for future situations. Karl Albrecht calls common sense *practical intelligence*. He defines it as "the mental ability to cope with the challenges and opportunities of life". He explains that common sense is situational, dependent on context, and that your common sense in one aspect of your life might be excellent while failing abysmally in another aspect of your life. As to the purpose of common sense, it is basically thinking that prevents you from making irrational mistakes or decisions, a thinking approach that may open your eyes to the possibility that insisting on being right prevents you from seeing the bigger picture.

- Common sense can also serve the purpose of removing you from being hidebound to rules, theories, ideas, and guidelines that would hamper or stifle the best decision in a particular situation. In other words, just because something says so, or just because it has always been done that way, is not a reason to abandon common sense about present needs and changed circumstances.

2. Understand the ease with which the human mind is convinced that an idea is right contrary to indicators clearly demonstrating otherwise.

We're human; we're fallible. And our brains work in certain ways as a means of providing shortcuts to ensure survival in a world where being chased by predators could end your life. In a modern world where caves and saber toothed tigers are no longer a constant companion, some of that reactive, split second judging can land us in hot water as we react instead of reflecting, assume instead of teasing apart the realities, and follow habit instead of challenging its continued utility. Some of the things our amazing mind is capable of doing to override common sense include:

- Maintaining our own sense of reality out of proportion with identifiable reality. While each of us creates a reality out of our own experiences and makes sense of our world through this personal lens, for the most part, we understand that our sense of reality is only a small portion of a much larger picture. For some people, however, their sense of reality becomes the only sense of reality and they believe that they can manipulate or magically transform situations to turn out the way they want them to be. In steps irrational behavior for some, and insanity for the less fortunate.
- Reflex or associative thinking. This is reactive thinking that is based simply on what we've learned through life, reenacting learned models and applying them to each new situation as it appears, *without* modifying the thought processes being applied. This type of thinking leads to errors in thinking because we refuse to push beyond standard associations formed in our

mind about how things "should be". When we apply what we know to a present situation by reference to a similar past situation by merely applying our mind's template without adjusting for the context, we're overriding common sense. Even where this template is a bad fit, the insistent or biased mind just ignores the parts of the template that don't fit by trimming them off mentally and only seeing the parts that "match". Hence, we have our problem solved without thinking it through. This type of thinking tends to make us easily swayed by current popular theories and fads, such as the current tendency in some societies to control social opinion through inflating fears of germs, criminals and terrorists, and job unavailability.

- Invoking absolute certainty. Absolutist black and white thinking about the world and others in it in a way that never allows space for doubt is often a cause for forgetting to apply common sense. For such a thinker, the "one true way" is the only way and therefore *seems* like common sense even though it isn't.
- Pigheadedness. A simple unwillingness to be wrong. Ever. Founded on any number of reasons including insecurities, fear, incomprehension, anger,

and fear of ridicule, pigheadedness is the cause of many an irrational and unjustifiable decision or action.

3. Divorce yourself from reality.

This isn't an invitation to insanity. This is a request to consider that *your* sense of reality isn't real. What you see is what you've programmed your brain to see. And once you start down the slippery slope of self-confirmation that reality is only ever what you see it as, you're open to the possibilities of bigotry, selfishness, intolerance, and prejudice because you'll constantly seek to make everyone and everything else conform to *your* standard of reality, and your standard of "what's right".[3] By divorcing yourself from this one-sided reality, and learning as much as you can about how other people perceive the world and our place in it, you begin to make room for common sense to grow because your sense is built on "common" experiences, not just your own.

- Start by taking a look at your own emotions, beliefs, and practices to make sure they're not overriding your common sense. Test different scenarios in your mind to try to ascertain the practical consequences of applying the decision or action the way you want to. Is it practical, have you accounted for everything, and what will happen if things go wrong? If things go

wrong, can you fix them and if you can't, what will be the consequences?
- Consult with others. If your reality is clouding your judgment too much, reach out and discuss the situation with others to gain wider appreciation of their perspectives and ideas. This is most important where you are too close to a situation and any decision or action you take might be infected by your proximity.

4. Acquaint yourself with your reflective mind.

This is the part of your thinking where true common sense resides. The part that takes a bit of time out from the cleverness, the brightness, the importance of everything rushing at you right now and suggests that it's time to add a dose of cold water to the excitement. Reflective intelligence is about being able to stand back and view the bigger picture so that you realistically appraise the situation or environment directly around you rather than forcing yourself to conform to its suitability or practicing wishful thinking. After an accurate appraisal of the situation, a reflective mindset enables you to set goals that are realistic given the parameters you're working within, and to take sensible actions toward meeting those goals. Daniel Willingham cites examples of people who throw money at the stock market, or people who choose unsuitable life situations as people who made decisions or took actions without using reflective thinking. Rationalizing that external signs seem fine while ignoring complete mismatches to the person you are or the beliefs you hold is a denial of common sense. In other words, just because other people do or use something effectively isn't a sign that it will suit you too; you need to put your own reflective mind to work on each situation to decide whether it will be a fit for you, your lifestyle, and those around you directly impacted by your decisions.

- Do less, think more. Siimon Reynolds says that many of us are suffering from "Obsessive Do-Itis". This simply means we're obsessed with doing more all the time instead of thinking. And while we're running around frantically being busy all the time, we're not being productive and we're contributing to a culture that admires incessantly busy people. Is this common sense? Hardly. It is about working harder and longer without taking time out to reflect.
- Allocate thinking time every single day, even if it's only 20 minutes. Siimon Reynolds suggests that you try this for one week, and says that at the end of it, you'll notice much reduced stress levels.[5] And your common sense will improve markedly.

5. Reacquaint yourself with your rapid cognition.

The previous step has just suggested that you need to reflect more before you take decisions or act. But the obvious flipside to reflection is the reality that some things need very fast thinking and rapid decisions that will produce sound results. Rapid cognition is the type of thinking that tells you that you're not going to connect with a person the moment that you meet them, or that a poorly placed ladder is going to fall sooner rather than later and needs to be shifted pronto, or that you need to quickly jump out of the way of an out-of-control car *now*. How do you marry rapid cognition to reflective thinking under the rubric of "common sense"? It's simple - spend your reflecting time wisely so that you will react wisely when quick thinking is required. Common sense builds on your reflection over past experiences, enabling you to refine your understanding of the world and how it works time and time again. This is in contrast to a person who only ever reacts on gut reactions, biases, and has failed to reflect on prior experiences. Reflection will bring about sound "gut reactions" or fast assessments of situations because your reaction is based on having taken the time to work through errors and successes of past experiences.

- Malcolm Gladwell says in *Blink* that "decisions made very quickly can be every bit as good as decisions made cautiously and deliberately".[6] The problem arises when we want something to be other than what it really is - falling back into our own idea of reality rather than the many realities around us. And that's when our common sense fails us.

6. Learn things that are basic common sense.

There are things that every human being should know how to do and not leave to another person, things that go to the heart of personal survival, self-knowledge, and long-term health and safety. In this way, you can learn common sense through practical knowledge and application, informing you accurately when times are harder or when you must react quickly.

- *Knowing how to cook and how the food gets to your table.* For every person who proudly proclaims that he or she does not know how to cook, there is a person easily persuaded by others that any food is suitable for them, no matter how unhealthy or how unethically or unproductively sourced. It's no badge of honor to not know how to cook for yourself; it's often a sign of laziness or a rebellion against supposed domesticity. Knowing how to cook is basic common sense because it will ensure your healthy survival under any conditions. And, no matter how

infrequently you use this skill, it's enjoyable and rewarding.
- *Knowing how to grow your own food.* Being able to grow your own food is an assurance of self-survival. Learn the skill if you haven't already and instill it in your kids.
- *Knowing about nutrition.* If you're cooking for yourself, and perhaps growing your own food, you'll be more connected with your body's need for healthy nutrition. Eat healthily most of the time, in moderation, and with an eye to meeting all appropriate nutritional needs for your age, gender, height, and personal conditions.
- *Knowing and respecting your surrounds.* Its common sense to know what local conditions impact your life, from weather to wildlife. Take the time to get to know your local environment and respond to it appropriately, from adequately weatherproofing your home to removing invasive species from your garden.
- *Knowing how to budget and not spend more than you're earning.* It's common sense to only spend what you have. Sadly, many people manage to forget this in an orgy of frequent over-spending, and behaving as if a bulging credit card debt came as a complete surprise to them. Over-spending is an irrational habit, as is hiding unopened bills at the back of a closet; reining in

the spending with a budget and self-restraint is common sense in action. And make sure to get all important financial decisions and agreements in writing, from loans to sales; you can never be too careful when it comes to money.
- *Knowing the limitations of your own body.* This includes knowing which foods wreak havoc with your body, which foods work for you, knowing how many hours of sleep you need, and knowing the type of exercise that benefits your body and metabolism best; read widely but figure out for yourself what harms and heals your body, as you're the real expert on this topic. Moreover, you're no superhero - ignoring bodily injuries is done at your own peril, such as continuing to carry heavy loads with an aching back, or refusing to acknowledge constant pains.
- *Knowing how to analyze situations and think for yourself.* Instead of digesting the pulp media thrown at you every day, and ending up in a state of fear because every second news item is a crime or disaster, start thinking about the reality behind the newsfeed and start thinking about life and happenings with a healthy, open, and questioning mindset. Help free others from the fear of media by teaching them how to recognize the tactics used.

- *Knowing how to repair items.* In a world heavily dependent on disposal of items rather than repairing them, we're adding to the Earth's burden. And, we're beholden to those who manufacture items with in-built obsolescence because we've lost the ability to tinker and fix things ourselves. Learning how to fix or mend clothes, appliances, household objects, car engines, and many other items that are important to our daily functioning, is not only liberating but is also an important way to exercise our common sense.
- *Knowing how to plan in advance.* So that you're not doing things haphazardly, more expensively, or without an idea of the consequences, learn to plan ahead. Forward thinking is always a sign of good common sense, as is being able to review the consequences of different outcomes.
- *Knowing how to be resourceful.* Resourcefulness is the art of "making do"; it's about taking small things and making them go a long way with a little imagination and elbow grease. It's about being able to thrive under difficult conditions and still prosper and not feel deprived. Resourcefulness is a key part of using common sense, and again, it's a skill that liberates you from consuming to live.
- *Knowing how to connect with community.* It's common sense to be a part of your community;

unfortunately many people prefer to bunker down and remain aloof or unhindered by the others around them. Connecting with others in your community is part of being human, of relating, and of opening yourself up to sharing and generosity.
- *Knowing how to keep safe.* Whether you're in public or at home, safety is a matter of common sense. Pushing saucepan handles away from you on the stove, looking both ways when crossing the street, walking with a friend or group in dark areas of the city at night instead of being alone, etc. All of these are common sense safety actions that can be planned for and put into action before anything harmful happens; and doing so will often avert problems altogether. Think prevention, not disaster.

7. Put new common sense thinking habits into place.

Take the philosophy, the psychology, and the popular theories behind how we think and add this understanding to the active ways in which you can use your common sense. Read How to think "outside of the box" to get some great ideas for restoring your sense of relying on your own innovative thinking processes. And Karl Albrecht suggests that the following methods will help to keep your practical

intelligence (common sense) in top shape (and it's recommended that you read his book in its entirety).
- Practice mental flexibility. This is the ability to stay open-minded and to listen to other people's notions and ideas, even if they scare you or derail your own thinking. It does you good to practice mental elasticity and to stretch yourself beyond the things you think you know already.
- Use affirmative thinking. This is the way of perceiving yourself and others in a positive manner, always looking to see the best in others and yourself, and making constant conscious decisions about who or what you will allow yourself to be influenced by, and what you will consider worthy of devoting your thinking time to. This isn't as simplistic as chanting affirmations or thinking happy thoughts; the mental work required to maintain an affirmative, conscious mindset is hard but rewarding.
- Rely on semantic sanity. This is about using language to support clear thinking freed from dogma.
- Value ideas. This concept leads you to accepting new ideas rather than immediately knocking them on the head as unfamiliar, insane, or undoable. How do you know they don't match your viewpoint until you've worked through them? Equally, valuing ideas encapsulates the need to reflect often, for without

adequate time for reflection, you'll fail to come up with your own ideas.

8. If you put in the constant hard yards of thinking things through carefully for yourself as well as learning all that you can about the world and other's thoughts about the world, you're well placed.

You don't have to be highly educated; you do have to be [open-minded](#) and curious. And realize that this is a process, not a destination. You will have to make the mental effort throughout your life as to which messages you absorb and which people you allow to influence your thinking. Even this article is but one source of guidance on common sense – analyze it, critique its applicability to your own circumstances, and cherry pick, discard, or adopt those things that suit you or don't fit with you. After all, doing so just makes plain common sense.

There you have it, an 8 step process to acquiring a common sense mentality. You now have the ingredients and the process to embrace. Will you choose common sense, and embrace the process? Or will you continue living a life based on tomfoolery and bad decisions? The choice is yours.

Phase II: Project Management - The Model

What is Project Management?

Project management involves planning and organization of a company's (Individual or Families) resources to move a specific task, event, or duty towards completion. It typically involves a one-time project rather than an ongoing activity, and resources managed include personnel, finances, technology, and intellectual property. A project manager (Head of household or Teacher) helps to define the goals and objectives of the project and determines when the various project components are to be completed and by whom; she/he also creates quality control checks to ensure completed components meet a certain standard.

The Project Management Model: 5 Phases of Project Management

1. Initiation - This is where all projects begin. The importance of the project is determined, as well as its feasibility (can it be done).

2. Planning - Once approved, a team is assembled (if needed) and you begin planning how to manage the project, and justify whether it makes sense.

3. Execution - Now that you have the plan, it's time to start the project. This is where the rubber hits the road, and you can't just cruise. You have to get moving, as most projects have time commitments.

4. Monitor & Control - To Ensure that the project plan is being actualized, all aspects of the project must be monitored and adjusted as needed.

5. Close - The Project isn't over once the project goals and objectives have been met. The last phase of the project is closing it out.

The Management Study Guide has this to say about The Importance of Project Management

Project management is the art of managing the project (Your Life) and its deliverables with a view to produce finished products or services (Life Outcomes). There are many ways in which a project can be carried out and the way in which it is executed is project management.

Project management includes: identifying requirements, establishing clear and achievable objectives, balancing the competing demands from the different stakeholders and ensuring that a commonality of purpose is achieved.

It is clear that unless there is a structured and scientific approach to the practice of management, organizations would find themselves adrift in the Ocean called organizational development and hence would be unable to meet the myriad challenges that the modern era throws at them. Hence, the importance of project management to organizations cannot be emphasized more and the succeeding paragraphs provide some reasons why organizations must take the practice of project management seriously.

Without a scientific approach to the task of managing the projects and achieving objectives, it would be very difficult for the organizations to successfully execute the projects within the constraints of time, scope and quality and deliver the required result. In other words, there has to be a framework and a defined way of doing things to ensure that there is a structure to the art of project management.

Thus, project management is about creating structure and managing the project commitments and the delivery of agreed upon results. By using the methods of project management as described in the PMBOK and allied technical journals, organizations can seek to achieve control over the project environment and ensure that the project deliverables are being managed. Managers face what is known as the "triple constraint". This is the competing demands of time, scope and quality upon the project manager's list of things to do and how well the project manager manages these constraints goes a long way in determining the success of the project. Without the use of Project Management, managers and organizations would find themselves facing an unpredictable and chaotic environment over which they have little control. Thus, Project Management is both necessary and essential to the success of the project.

Project Management is too big an area to be covered in a few pages and the attempt is to provide concise and lucid definitions of the various terms and terminologies associated with a project. It is important to note that project management provides a framework within which subsequent actions by the organization can be taken and in this way, it is essential for organizations to adopt the framework provided by the practice of project management.

Conclusion

In conclusion, Project Management and the practice of the same have become indispensable to the modern day project manager and they form the basis of much of what is achieved during the course of a project. Thus, the idea of a project being managed professionally lends itself to the concepts and processes laid out for the practitioners of the art of Project Management.

Basically, in life most everything we do can be looked at as a project, and you have just been given a process by which you can proceed in life and finish what you start. What's your next project? **It should be YOURSELF…**

Phase III: Accountability – Own Your Actions

Webster defines Accountability as follows:

The Quality of being accountable; an obligation or willingness to accept responsibility or to account for one's actions.

Remember as you choose your Behaviors, you also choose your Consequences

If you will hold yourself accountable for your actions, responsibilities, and goals, you can achieve anything that is important to you.

By choosing to become accountable you have taken the first step in your maturation. Instead of having excuses for your recklessness, plain and simply own up to it and you will find that people are far more forgiving. Tell lies and no one will be there for you. We have to be able to look ourselves in the mirror and respect the individual we see. It begins there; as if you can't be honest with your reflection you probably can't be honest with others. Show up and put in quality time and you will see that quality time and respect will be given in return.

Showing Up: The Importance of Just Showing Up

You can say no anytime you want—but if you say yes, then mean it and show up and fulfill your commitment.

Woody Allen said 80 percent of success is showing up. However don't just show up, participate. You know what I mean. You can't *just* go to class. You have to actually pay attention, ask questions, engage with the material, do the homework, understand what's going on, study smart, meet with the teacher, and do well on the exams— or at least some mixture of these things.

Accountability has to become personal, and we must all learn to own it if we are to advance in this life. It is no easy task to become accountable, however it is the best and most respected way to live.

Personal Accountability – A requirement for Life Advancement: By Todd Smith

Accountability is normally viewed as being responsible—giving an explanation of your actions—to somebody for something. However, today's lesson is not about someone holding you accountable. It's about you holding yourself accountable.

When you take 100 percent responsibility for holding yourself accountable, your performance will improve, your relationships will flourish, your market value will soar, people's respect for you will skyrocket, you will be a great example for others to follow, and your self-esteem will grow.

How is it that in all these areas of your life you can see such dramatic improvement? Because when you hold yourself accountable to doing the things you know you should do, you will distinguish yourself from the crowd.

I am convinced if you want to advance your life personally or professionally, you must hold yourself accountable for your actions, responsibilities, and goals. Think about it. Why should it be someone else's job to make sure you are doing the things that you know you should to be doing?

The mindset I adopted more than 25 years ago is this: *it is up to me and no one else to make sure I am doing what I know I should be doing*. When someone has to hold me accountable, because I failed to do what I should have done, I have a serious conversation with myself. My belief is that *no one* should have to hold me accountable for my actions, responsibilities and goals. While I appreciate others helping me get better, I am the one that must hold myself to a high standard.

Some feel that there are 3 types of accountability. Let's have a look at the 3 areas in which you must hold yourself accountable.

1. Your actions and choices—this would include such things as:
- The way in which you communicate with others
- How you spend your time
- Your behavior and manners
- The consideration and respect you show others
- Your eating habits and exercising routine
- Your attitude and thoughts
- The way you respond to challenges

2. Your responsibilities—this would include these types of things:
- Returning calls, emails, and texts in a timely manner
- Being on time for business and personal appointments
- Keeping your home, car, and workplace clean
- Spending less than you earn
- Doing the things you agreed to do when you agreed to do them
- Executing your job description to the best of your ability
- Writing things down on a "To Do" list so you don't forget

3. Your goals—this would include your:
- Fitness and health targets
- Financial goals
- Family objectives
- Career ambitions
- Personal goals
- Marital enhancement
- Any other goals you have set for yourself

Make no mistake about it. You cannot achieve any worthwhile personal or professional goal, if you don't hold yourself accountable. The reason is simple. It's your life! If you have to be held accountable at work, don't expect to be promoted or to experience any type of significant career advancement. If you have to be held accountable at home by your parents, roommate or spouse, it will grow old fast and your relationships will deteriorate.

Holding YOURSELF accountable is nothing more than following through with YOUR commitments and responsibilities. It's doing what YOU know YOU should do, when YOU should do it. Whether YOU are 15 years old or 60 years old, let today be the day that YOU make the commitment to YOURSELF that YOU will NEVER again require anyone else to hold YOU accountable. Let me also encourage you to start keeping a prioritized "To Do" list and focus on holding yourself accountable to working through your tasks in a prioritized sequence. This is your life, take control and be responsible for it. As always there will be exceptions, so if you are struggling with personal accountability and need the help of others I strongly encourage you to seek it out. Now, are you ready to become more accountable? Then let's get started.

Phase IV - Health & Recreation - Keeping Active

Why Live Healthy?

A healthy lifestyle involves eating a balanced diet, exercising regularly and managing stress effectively. Making these healthy choices every day can affect more than your physical appearance -- it can also increase both the length and quality of your life by boosting your immunity to disease and keeping you emotionally healthy.

Creates More Energy and Stamina

Health is more than the absence of illness. A healthy body rewards you with a lifetime of service in the form of high energy levels, strength and longevity. According to Science Daily, low-intensity exercise can decrease fatigue by 65 percent while boosting energy levels up to 20 percent. Healthy adults should aim for 30 minutes of moderate-intensity aerobic exercise each day for optimal fitness. Activity can be spread throughout the day and may include small changes like parking further from entrances or taking the stairs instead of the elevator.

Helps Disease Prevention

Chronic diseases like heart disease, type II diabetes and cancer are endemic in today's society. While risk factors like family history are uncontrollable, lifestyle factors such as diet, exercise and avoidance of harmful habits can go a long way toward preventing disease. The Mayo Clinic states that eating a diet low in saturated fat, exercising for 30 minutes daily and avoiding tobacco use greatly reduce the risk of heart disease — the most common chronic disease in the United States. Eating a nutritious diet and exercising regularly may also help prevent cancer development in people with an increased genetic risk for the disease, according to the American Cancer Society.

Adds to Your Beauty and Appearance

Healthy lifestyle habits are vital for maintaining a youthful, attractive appearance. For example, vitamin A supports healthy skin, hair and nails, while antioxidants like vitamin C and selenium help prevent free radical damage involved in the aging process. Healthy lifestyle choices like eating a balanced diet and exercising regularly also help prevent obesity. Avoiding excessive sun exposure, smoking and other potentially harmful habits promotes a youthful appearance by protecting against damage that can accelerate the aging of your skin.

Remember Community Service

To truly strive for a healthy lifestyle we must learn to give back to the very communities in which we reside. We have to adopt a sustainability mentality and explore ways to use our natural resources without destroying the ecological balance of our community. Whether its community gardening, volunteering at a local non-profit, or just sitting with an elderly neighbor, we've got to always have a hand to those less fortunate and show that we possess the very milk of human kindness needed to assist others.

Wow, the areas that are spoken to here are basically the staples for living a long healthy prosperous life, as it's the healthy, good looking, and eager folks that always seem to succeed. Get up, get out, and get moving if you wish to aspire to greatness. Look at all the great ones, Michael Jordan, Roger Federer, Serena Williams, and I am sure you see where I'm going with this. To be great you have to dream big, and be willing to shoot for the stars.

Now how do you achieve this goal? You achieve this goal by staying healthy, staying active, staying hungry, making adjustments, and holding yourself accountable to this 5 Phase System for Living. Be great every day, and when you get the chance always choose to **Dance….**

Phase V: My Main Ingredient

Do you have one?

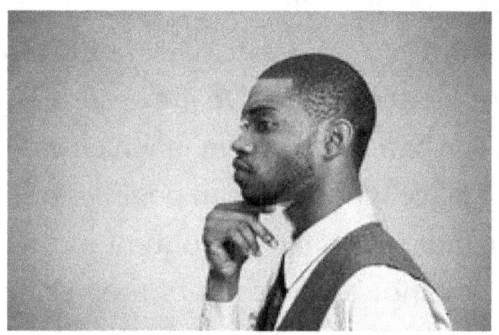

Think About it…..

To find out what my main Ingredient is, catch me at one of my motivational speaking presentations. We all need one, and I absolutely refuse to live without mine. Live life, and never stop learning.

The Decision

So here we are, and you decided to read The System. I know what you're thinking, you're either saying this is a bunch of nonsense or you're going to give it a try. If you think it's nonsense, then just walk away and nothing will change. However if you are up to the **challenge**, and you choose to live life the right way then make the decision to live life according to this **Blueprint** and the very **System** in which we live in becomes a place where we can begin to honestly and truly judge individuals by the content of their character, and not by the color of their skin as spoken by the late great Dr. Martin Luther King Jr.

Now if you are still reading and I pray that you are, I offer you my support, and I know that you have what it takes to persevere. I once heard a preacher articulate "you can't lead where you don't go, and you can't teach what you don't know. By making **The System** your way of life you will be passing on this **Blueprint** to all those that come after you. The philosophy is known as Reach One Teach One. Let's get started.

Bibliography

Wiki Now; How to Develop Common Sense

ProjectManager.com; Phases of Project Management.

Smith, Todd; Personal Accountability – A requirement for Life Advancement.

Definitions of System, Common Sense, Process and Accountability; Merriam Webster Dictionary

The Creator of The System
Rick James McPhearson

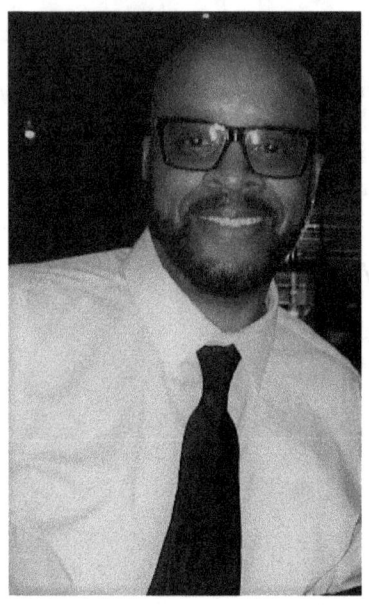

I wish **The System** were around when I grew up, as I know it would've been a beneficial tool for my boys and me. On the other hand you have this tool right before you, so my question to you is; are you going to use it? I truly believe that life holds a different opportunity for each of us. **Go Boldly Into Yours My Friend….**

To contact Rick, or have him come out to speak send your email message to:
rick.mcphearson@thesactofoundation.org

Write Your Questions Here

1.

2.

3.

4.

5.

6.

7.

8.

Use this section to take notes:

Notes continued

Use this section to write Your Blueprint

Your Blueprint Continued...

www.ingramcontent.com/pod-product-compliance
Lightning Source LLC
Chambersburg PA
CBHW071417290426
44108CB00014B/1858